I0840315

COVID-19
Track and Trace
DIARY

Name	
Telephone	
Date From	
Date To	

As we come out of lockdown and venture back into the COVID-19 version of normal, now more than ever it is essential to know where you have been, when and with whom. Despite taking the precautions of social distancing and wearing a face covering, if you get the telephone call, can you be sure when and where you were?

Don't guess, track it in this useful diary. Contains 62 pages, with three location entries per page, allowing you to record:

- Date
- Location - where you were, where you went
- Time
- Who you were with - friends, family or on your own
- Who you encountered - a few people, socially distancing or crowds, not socially distancing

Take care. Stay safe!

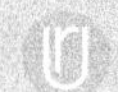

Published by Really Useful Publishing Company
Publisher's Cataloguing–in–Publication data

Webster, David
A title of book: *COVID-19 Track and Trace Diary* / David Webster

The names and/or references to any organisation, operator, manufacturer, supplier, product, service, brand etc appearing in this book are the trademarks and/or registered trademarks of their respective owners. They are used for illustrative purposes only and do not imply any endorsement, recommendation or association.

E&OE First Edition, July 2020   ISBN: 978-1-71676-012-9

Cover Image by Tumisu at www.pixabay.com

Day	Date	Month	Year

Location *shop, store etc*	
Time From	
Time To	
With *family, friends etc*	
Near *other shoppers etc*	

Day	Date	Month	Year

Location *shop, store etc*	
Time From	
Time To	
With *family, friends etc*	
Near *other shoppers etc*	

Day	Date	Month	Year

Location *shop, store etc*	
Time From	
Time To	
With *family, friends etc*	
Near *other shoppers etc*	

Day	Date	Month	Year

Location shop, store etc	
Time From	
Time To	
With family, friends etc	
Near other shoppers etc	

Day	Date	Month	Year

Location shop, store etc	
Time From	
Time To	
With family, friends etc	
Near other shoppers etc	

Day	Date	Month	Year

Location shop, store etc	
Time From	
Time To	
With family, friends etc	
Near other shoppers etc	

Day	Date	Month	Year

Location *shop, store etc*	
Time From	
Time To	
With *family, friends etc*	
Near *other shoppers etc*	

Day	Date	Month	Year

Location *shop, store etc*	
Time From	
Time To	
With *family, friends etc*	
Near *other shoppers etc*	

Day	Date	Month	Year

Location *shop, store etc*	
Time From	
Time To	
With *family, friends etc*	
Near *other shoppers etc*	

Day	Date	Month	Year

Location *shop, store etc*	
Time From	
Time To	
With *family, friends etc*	
Near *other shoppers etc*	

Day	Date	Month	Year

Location *shop, store etc*	
Time From	
Time To	
With *family, friends etc*	
Near *other shoppers etc*	

Day	Date	Month	Year

Location *shop, store etc*	
Time From	
Time To	
With *family, friends etc*	
Near *other shoppers etc*	

Day	Date	Month	Year

Location *shop, store etc*	
Time From	
Time To	
With *family, friends etc*	
Near *other shoppers etc*	

Day	Date	Month	Year

Location *shop, store etc*	
Time From	
Time To	
With *family, friends etc*	
Near *other shoppers etc*	

Day	Date	Month	Year

Location *shop, store etc*	
Time From	
Time To	
With *family, friends etc*	
Near *other shoppers etc*	

Day	Date	Month	Year

Location *shop, store etc*	
Time From	
Time To	
With *family, friends etc*	
Near *other shoppers etc*	

Day	Date	Month	Year

Location *shop, store etc*	
Time From	
Time To	
With *family, friends etc*	
Near *other shoppers etc*	

Day	Date	Month	Year

Location *shop, store etc*	
Time From	
Time To	
With *family, friends etc*	
Near *other shoppers etc*	

Day	Date	Month	Year

Location *shop, store etc*	
Time From	
Time To	
With *family, friends etc*	
Near *other shoppers etc*	

Day	Date	Month	Year

Location *shop, store etc*	
Time From	
Time To	
With *family, friends etc*	
Near *other shoppers etc*	

Day	Date	Month	Year

Location *shop, store etc*	
Time From	
Time To	
With *family, friends etc*	
Near *other shoppers etc*	

Day	Date	Month	Year

Location shop, store etc	
Time From	
Time To	
With family, friends etc	
Near other shoppers etc	

Day	Date	Month	Year

Location shop, store etc	
Time From	
Time To	
With family, friends etc	
Near other shoppers etc	

Day	Date	Month	Year

Location shop, store etc	
Time From	
Time To	
With family, friends etc	
Near other shoppers etc	

Day	Date	Month	Year
Location *shop, store etc*			
Time From			
Time To			
With *family, friends etc*			
Near *other shoppers etc*			

Day	Date	Month	Year
Location *shop, store etc*			
Time From			
Time To			
With *family, friends etc*			
Near *other shoppers etc*			

Day	Date	Month	Year
Location *shop, store etc*			
Time From			
Time To			
With *family, friends etc*			
Near *other shoppers etc*			

Day	Date	Month	Year

Location *shop, store etc*	
Time From	
Time To	
With *family, friends etc*	
Near *other shoppers etc*	

Day	Date	Month	Year

Location *shop, store etc*	
Time From	
Time To	
With *family, friends etc*	
Near *other shoppers etc*	

Day	Date	Month	Year

Location *shop, store etc*	
Time From	
Time To	
With *family, friends etc*	
Near *other shoppers etc*	

Day	Date	Month	Year

Location *shop, store etc*	
Time From	
Time To	
With *family, friends etc*	
Near *other shoppers etc*	

Day	Date	Month	Year

Location *shop, store etc*	
Time From	
Time To	
With *family, friends etc*	
Near *other shoppers etc*	

Day	Date	Month	Year

Location *shop, store etc*	
Time From	
Time To	
With *family, friends etc*	
Near *other shoppers etc*	

Day	Date	Month	Year

Location *shop, store etc*	
Time From	
Time To	
With *family, friends etc*	
Near *other shoppers etc*	

Day	Date	Month	Year

Location *shop, store etc*	
Time From	
Time To	
With *family, friends etc*	
Near *other shoppers etc*	

Day	Date	Month	Year

Location *shop, store etc*	
Time From	
Time To	
With *family, friends etc*	
Near *other shoppers etc*	

Day	Date	Month	Year

Location *shop, store etc*	
Time From	
Time To	
With *family, friends etc*	
Near *other shoppers etc*	

Day	Date	Month	Year

Location *shop, store etc*	
Time From	
Time To	
With *family, friends etc*	
Near *other shoppers etc*	

Day	Date	Month	Year

Location *shop, store etc*	
Time From	
Time To	
With *family, friends etc*	
Near *other shoppers etc*	

Day	Date	Month	Year

Location *shop, store etc*	
Time From	
Time To	
With *family, friends etc*	
Near *other shoppers etc*	

Day	Date	Month	Year

Location *shop, store etc*	
Time From	
Time To	
With *family, friends etc*	
Near *other shoppers etc*	

Day	Date	Month	Year

Location *shop, store etc*	
Time From	
Time To	
With *family, friends etc*	
Near *other shoppers etc*	

Day	Date	Month	Year

Location shop, store etc	
Time From	
Time To	
With family, friends etc	
Near other shoppers etc	

Day	Date	Month	Year

Location shop, store etc	
Time From	
Time To	
With family, friends etc	
Near other shoppers etc	

Day	Date	Month	Year

Location shop, store etc	
Time From	
Time To	
With family, friends etc	
Near other shoppers etc	

Day	Date	Month	Year

Location *shop, store etc*	
Time From	
Time To	
With *family, friends etc*	
Near *other shoppers etc*	

Day	Date	Month	Year

Location *shop, store etc*	
Time From	
Time To	
With *family, friends etc*	
Near *other shoppers etc*	

Day	Date	Month	Year

Location *shop, store etc*	
Time From	
Time To	
With *family, friends etc*	
Near *other shoppers etc*	

Day	Date	Month	Year

Location *shop, store etc*	
Time From	
Time To	
With *family, friends etc*	
Near *other shoppers etc*	

Day	Date	Month	Year

Location *shop, store etc*	
Time From	
Time To	
With *family, friends etc*	
Near *other shoppers etc*	

Day	Date	Month	Year

Location *shop, store etc*	
Time From	
Time To	
With *family, friends etc*	
Near *other shoppers etc*	

Day	Date	Month	Year

Location *shop, store etc*	
Time From	
Time To	
With *family, friends etc*	
Near *other shoppers etc*	

Day	Date	Month	Year

Location *shop, store etc*	
Time From	
Time To	
With *family, friends etc*	
Near *other shoppers etc*	

Day	Date	Month	Year

Location *shop, store etc*	
Time From	
Time To	
With *family, friends etc*	
Near *other shoppers etc*	

Day	Date	Month	Year

Location *shop, store etc*	
Time From	
Time To	
With *family, friends etc*	
Near *other shoppers etc*	

Day	Date	Month	Year

Location *shop, store etc*	
Time From	
Time To	
With *family, friends etc*	
Near *other shoppers etc*	

Day	Date	Month	Year

Location *shop, store etc*	
Time From	
Time To	
With *family, friends etc*	
Near *other shoppers etc*	

Day	Date	Month	Year

Location *shop, store etc*	
Time From	
Time To	
With *family, friends etc*	
Near *other shoppers etc*	

Day	Date	Month	Year

Location *shop, store etc*	
Time From	
Time To	
With *family, friends etc*	
Near *other shoppers etc*	

Day	Date	Month	Year

Location *shop, store etc*	
Time From	
Time To	
With *family, friends etc*	
Near *other shoppers etc*	

Day	Date	Month	Year

Location *shop, store etc*	
Time From	
Time To	
With *family, friends etc*	
Near *other shoppers etc*	

Day	Date	Month	Year

Location *shop, store etc*	
Time From	
Time To	
With *family, friends etc*	
Near *other shoppers etc*	

Day	Date	Month	Year

Location *shop, store etc*	
Time From	
Time To	
With *family, friends etc*	
Near *other shoppers etc*	

Day	Date	Month	Year

Location *shop, store etc*	
Time From	
Time To	
With *family, friends etc*	
Near *other shoppers etc*	

Day	Date	Month	Year

Location *shop, store etc*	
Time From	
Time To	
With *family, friends etc*	
Near *other shoppers etc*	

Day	Date	Month	Year

Location *shop, store etc*	
Time From	
Time To	
With *family, friends etc*	
Near *other shoppers etc*	

Day	Date	Month	Year

Location shop, store etc	
Time From	
Time To	
With family, friends etc	
Near other shoppers etc	

Day	Date	Month	Year

Location shop, store etc	
Time From	
Time To	
With family, friends etc	
Near other shoppers etc	

Day	Date	Month	Year

Location shop, store etc	
Time From	
Time To	
With family, friends etc	
Near other shoppers etc	

Day	Date	Month	Year

Location *shop, store etc*	
Time From	
Time To	
With *family, friends etc*	
Near *other shoppers etc*	

Day	Date	Month	Year

Location *shop, store etc*	
Time From	
Time To	
With *family, friends etc*	
Near *other shoppers etc*	

Day	Date	Month	Year

Location *shop, store etc*	
Time From	
Time To	
With *family, friends etc*	
Near *other shoppers etc*	

Day	Date	Month	Year

Location *shop, store etc*	
Time From	
Time To	
With *family, friends etc*	
Near *other shoppers etc*	

Day	Date	Month	Year

Location *shop, store etc*	
Time From	
Time To	
With *family, friends etc*	
Near *other shoppers etc*	

Day	Date	Month	Year

Location *shop, store etc*	
Time From	
Time To	
With *family, friends etc*	
Near *other shoppers etc*	

Day	Date	Month	Year

Location *shop, store etc*	
Time From	
Time To	
With *family, friends etc*	
Near *other shoppers etc*	

Day	Date	Month	Year

Location *shop, store etc*	
Time From	
Time To	
With *family, friends etc*	
Near *other shoppers etc*	

Day	Date	Month	Year

Location *shop, store etc*	
Time From	
Time To	
With *family, friends etc*	
Near *other shoppers etc*	

Day	Date	Month	Year

Location shop, store etc	
Time From	
Time To	
With family, friends etc	
Near other shoppers etc	

Day	Date	Month	Year

Location shop, store etc	
Time From	
Time To	
With family, friends etc	
Near other shoppers etc	

Day	Date	Month	Year

Location shop, store etc	
Time From	
Time To	
With family, friends etc	
Near other shoppers etc	

Day	Date	Month	Year

Location *shop, store etc*	
Time From	
Time To	
With *family, friends etc*	
Near *other shoppers etc*	

Day	Date	Month	Year

Location *shop, store etc*	
Time From	
Time To	
With *family, friends etc*	
Near *other shoppers etc*	

Day	Date	Month	Year

Location *shop, store etc*	
Time From	
Time To	
With *family, friends etc*	
Near *other shoppers etc*	

Day	Date	Month	Year

Location shop, store etc	
Time From	
Time To	
With family, friends etc	
Near other shoppers etc	

Day	Date	Month	Year

Location shop, store etc	
Time From	
Time To	
With family, friends etc	
Near other shoppers etc	

Day	Date	Month	Year

Location shop, store etc	
Time From	
Time To	
With family, friends etc	
Near other shoppers etc	

Day	Date	Month	Year

Location *shop, store etc*	
Time From	
Time To	
With *family, friends etc*	
Near *other shoppers etc*	

Day	Date	Month	Year

Location *shop, store etc*	
Time From	
Time To	
With *family, friends etc*	
Near *other shoppers etc*	

Day	Date	Month	Year

Location *shop, store etc*	
Time From	
Time To	
With *family, friends etc*	
Near *other shoppers etc*	

Day	Date	Month	Year

Location *shop, store etc*	
Time From	
Time To	
With *family, friends etc*	
Near *other shoppers etc*	

Day	Date	Month	Year

Location *shop, store etc*	
Time From	
Time To	
With *family, friends etc*	
Near *other shoppers etc*	

Day	Date	Month	Year

Location *shop, store etc*	
Time From	
Time To	
With *family, friends etc*	
Near *other shoppers etc*	

Day	Date	Month	Year

Location *shop, store etc*	
Time From	
Time To	
With *family, friends etc*	
Near *other shoppers etc*	

Day	Date	Month	Year

Location *shop, store etc*	
Time From	
Time To	
With *family, friends etc*	
Near *other shoppers etc*	

Day	Date	Month	Year

Location *shop, store etc*	
Time From	
Time To	
With *family, friends etc*	
Near *other shoppers etc*	

Day	Date	Month	Year
Location *shop, store etc*			
Time From			
Time To			
With *family, friends etc*			
Near *other shoppers etc*			

Day	Date	Month	Year
Location *shop, store etc*			
Time From			
Time To			
With *family, friends etc*			
Near *other shoppers etc*			

Day	Date	Month	Year
Location *shop, store etc*			
Time From			
Time To			
With *family, friends etc*			
Near *other shoppers etc*			

Day	Date	Month	Year

Location shop, store etc	
Time From	
Time To	
With family, friends etc	
Near other shoppers etc	

Day	Date	Month	Year

Location shop, store etc	
Time From	
Time To	
With family, friends etc	
Near other shoppers etc	

Day	Date	Month	Year

Location shop, store etc	
Time From	
Time To	
With family, friends etc	
Near other shoppers etc	

Day	Date	Month	Year
Location *shop, store etc*			
Time From			
Time To			
With *family, friends etc*			
Near *other shoppers etc*			

Day	Date	Month	Year
Location *shop, store etc*			
Time From			
Time To			
With *family, friends etc*			
Near *other shoppers etc*			

Day	Date	Month	Year
Location *shop, store etc*			
Time From			
Time To			
With *family, friends etc*			
Near *other shoppers etc*			

Day	Date	Month	Year

Location *shop, store etc*	
Time From	
Time To	
With *family, friends etc*	
Near *other shoppers etc*	

Day	Date	Month	Year

Location *shop, store etc*	
Time From	
Time To	
With *family, friends etc*	
Near *other shoppers etc*	

Day	Date	Month	Year

Location *shop, store etc*	
Time From	
Time To	
With *family, friends etc*	
Near *other shoppers etc*	

Day	Date	Month	Year
Location *shop, store etc*			
Time From			
Time To			
With *family, friends etc*			
Near *other shoppers etc*			

Day	Date	Month	Year
Location *shop, store etc*			
Time From			
Time To			
With *family, friends etc*			
Near *other shoppers etc*			

Day	Date	Month	Year
Location *shop, store etc*			
Time From			
Time To			
With *family, friends etc*			
Near *other shoppers etc*			

Day	Date	Month	Year

Location *shop, store etc*	
Time From	
Time To	
With *family, friends etc*	
Near *other shoppers etc*	

Day	Date	Month	Year

Location *shop, store etc*	
Time From	
Time To	
With *family, friends etc*	
Near *other shoppers etc*	

Day	Date	Month	Year

Location *shop, store etc*	
Time From	
Time To	
With *family, friends etc*	
Near *other shoppers etc*	

Day	Date	Month	Year

Location *shop, store etc*	
Time From	
Time To	
With *family, friends etc*	
Near *other shoppers etc*	

Day	Date	Month	Year

Location *shop, store etc*	
Time From	
Time To	
With *family, friends etc*	
Near *other shoppers etc*	

Day	Date	Month	Year

Location *shop, store etc*	
Time From	
Time To	
With *family, friends etc*	
Near *other shoppers etc*	

Day	Date	Month	Year

Location *shop, store etc*	
Time From	
Time To	
With *family, friends etc*	
Near *other shoppers etc*	

Day	Date	Month	Year

Location *shop, store etc*	
Time From	
Time To	
With *family, friends etc*	
Near *other shoppers etc*	

Day	Date	Month	Year

Location *shop, store etc*	
Time From	
Time To	
With *family, friends etc*	
Near *other shoppers etc*	

Day	Date	Month	Year

Location *shop, store etc*	
Time From	
Time To	
With *family, friends etc*	
Near *other shoppers etc*	

Day	Date	Month	Year

Location *shop, store etc*	
Time From	
Time To	
With *family, friends etc*	
Near *other shoppers etc*	

Day	Date	Month	Year

Location *shop, store etc*	
Time From	
Time To	
With *family, friends etc*	
Near *other shoppers etc*	

Day	Date	Month	Year

Location *shop, store etc*	
Time From	
Time To	
With *family, friends etc*	
Near *other shoppers etc*	

Day	Date	Month	Year

Location *shop, store etc*	
Time From	
Time To	
With *family, friends etc*	
Near *other shoppers etc*	

Day	Date	Month	Year

Location *shop, store etc*	
Time From	
Time To	
With *family, friends etc*	
Near *other shoppers etc*	

Day	Date	Month	Year
Location *shop, store etc*			
Time From			
Time To			
With *family, friends etc*			
Near *other shoppers etc*			

Day	Date	Month	Year
Location *shop, store etc*			
Time From			
Time To			
With *family, friends etc*			
Near *other shoppers etc*			

Day	Date	Month	Year
Location *shop, store etc*			
Time From			
Time To			
With *family, friends etc*			
Near *other shoppers etc*			

Day	Date	Month	Year

Location *shop, store etc*	
Time From	
Time To	
With *family, friends etc*	
Near *other shoppers etc*	

Day	Date	Month	Year

Location *shop, store etc*	
Time From	
Time To	
With *family, friends etc*	
Near *other shoppers etc*	

Day	Date	Month	Year

Location *shop, store etc*	
Time From	
Time To	
With *family, friends etc*	
Near *other shoppers etc*	

Day	Date	Month	Year

Location shop, store etc	
Time From	
Time To	
With family, friends etc	
Near other shoppers etc	

Day	Date	Month	Year

Location shop, store etc	
Time From	
Time To	
With family, friends etc	
Near other shoppers etc	

Day	Date	Month	Year

Location shop, store etc	
Time From	
Time To	
With family, friends etc	
Near other shoppers etc	

Day	Date	Month	Year

Location *shop, store etc*	
Time From	
Time To	
With *family, friends etc*	
Near *other shoppers etc*	

Day	Date	Month	Year

Location *shop, store etc*	
Time From	
Time To	
With *family, friends etc*	
Near *other shoppers etc*	

Day	Date	Month	Year

Location *shop, store etc*	
Time From	
Time To	
With *family, friends etc*	
Near *other shoppers etc*	

Day	Date	Month	Year

Location *shop, store etc*	
Time From	
Time To	
With *family, friends etc*	
Near *other shoppers etc*	

Day	Date	Month	Year

Location *shop, store etc*	
Time From	
Time To	
With *family, friends etc*	
Near *other shoppers etc*	

Day	Date	Month	Year

Location *shop, store etc*	
Time From	
Time To	
With *family, friends etc*	
Near *other shoppers etc*	

Day	Date	Month	Year

Location *shop, store etc*	
Time From	
Time To	
With *family, friends etc*	
Near *other shoppers etc*	

Day	Date	Month	Year

Location *shop, store etc*	
Time From	
Time To	
With *family, friends etc*	
Near *other shoppers etc*	

Day	Date	Month	Year

Location *shop, store etc*	
Time From	
Time To	
With *family, friends etc*	
Near *other shoppers etc*	

Day	Date	Month	Year
Location *shop, store etc*			
Time From			
Time To			
With *family, friends etc*			
Near *other shoppers etc*			

Day	Date	Month	Year
Location *shop, store etc*			
Time From			
Time To			
With *family, friends etc*			
Near *other shoppers etc*			

Day	Date	Month	Year
Location *shop, store etc*			
Time From			
Time To			
With *family, friends etc*			
Near *other shoppers etc*			

Day	Date	Month	Year

Location *shop, store etc*	
Time From	
Time To	
With *family, friends etc*	
Near *other shoppers etc*	

Day	Date	Month	Year

Location *shop, store etc*	
Time From	
Time To	
With *family, friends etc*	
Near *other shoppers etc*	

Day	Date	Month	Year

Location *shop, store etc*	
Time From	
Time To	
With *family, friends etc*	
Near *other shoppers etc*	

Day	Date	Month	Year

Location *shop, store etc*	
Time From	
Time To	
With *family, friends etc*	
Near *other shoppers etc*	

Day	Date	Month	Year

Location *shop, store etc*	
Time From	
Time To	
With *family, friends etc*	
Near *other shoppers etc*	

Day	Date	Month	Year

Location *shop, store etc*	
Time From	
Time To	
With *family, friends etc*	
Near *other shoppers etc*	

Day	Date	Month	Year

Location *shop, store etc*	
Time From	
Time To	
With *family, friends etc*	
Near *other shoppers etc*	

Day	Date	Month	Year

Location *shop, store etc*	
Time From	
Time To	
With *family, friends etc*	
Near *other shoppers etc*	

Day	Date	Month	Year

Location *shop, store etc*	
Time From	
Time To	
With *family, friends etc*	
Near *other shoppers etc*	

Day	Date	Month	Year

Location *shop, store etc*	
Time From	
Time To	
With *family, friends etc*	
Near *other shoppers etc*	

Day	Date	Month	Year

Location *shop, store etc*	
Time From	
Time To	
With *family, friends etc*	
Near *other shoppers etc*	

Day	Date	Month	Year

Location *shop, store etc*	
Time From	
Time To	
With *family, friends etc*	
Near *other shoppers etc*	

Day	Date	Month	Year

Location shop, store etc	
Time From	
Time To	
With family, friends etc	
Near other shoppers etc	

Day	Date	Month	Year

Location shop, store etc	
Time From	
Time To	
With family, friends etc	
Near other shoppers etc	

Day	Date	Month	Year

Location shop, store etc	
Time From	
Time To	
With family, friends etc	
Near other shoppers etc	

Day	Date	Month	Year

Location *shop, store etc*	
Time From	
Time To	
With *family, friends etc*	
Near *other shoppers etc*	

Day	Date	Month	Year

Location *shop, store etc*	
Time From	
Time To	
With *family, friends etc*	
Near *other shoppers etc*	

Day	Date	Month	Year

Location *shop, store etc*	
Time From	
Time To	
With *family, friends etc*	
Near *other shoppers etc*	

Day	Date	Month	Year

Location *shop, store etc*	
Time From	
Time To	
With *family, friends etc*	
Near *other shoppers etc*	

Day	Date	Month	Year

Location *shop, store etc*	
Time From	
Time To	
With *family, friends etc*	
Near *other shoppers etc*	

Day	Date	Month	Year

Location *shop, store etc*	
Time From	
Time To	
With *family, friends etc*	
Near *other shoppers etc*	

Day	Date	Month	Year
Location shop, store etc			
Time From			
Time To			
With family, friends etc			
Near other shoppers etc			

Day	Date	Month	Year
Location shop, store etc			
Time From			
Time To			
With family, friends etc			
Near other shoppers etc			

Day	Date	Month	Year
Location shop, store etc			
Time From			
Time To			
With family, friends etc			
Near other shoppers etc			

Day	Date	Month	Year

Location *shop, store etc*	
Time From	
Time To	
With *family, friends etc*	
Near *other shoppers etc*	

Day	Date	Month	Year

Location *shop, store etc*	
Time From	
Time To	
With *family, friends etc*	
Near *other shoppers etc*	

Day	Date	Month	Year

Location *shop, store etc*	
Time From	
Time To	
With *family, friends etc*	
Near *other shoppers etc*	

Day	Date	Month	Year

Location *shop, store etc*	
Time From	
Time To	
With *family, friends etc*	
Near *other shoppers etc*	

Day	Date	Month	Year

Location *shop, store etc*	
Time From	
Time To	
With *family, friends etc*	
Near *other shoppers etc*	

Day	Date	Month	Year

Location *shop, store etc*	
Time From	
Time To	
With *family, friends etc*	
Near *other shoppers etc*	

Day	Date	Month	Year

Location *shop, store etc*	
Time From	
Time To	
With *family, friends etc*	
Near *other shoppers etc*	

Day	Date	Month	Year

Location *shop, store etc*	
Time From	
Time To	
With *family, friends etc*	
Near *other shoppers etc*	

Day	Date	Month	Year

Location *shop, store etc*	
Time From	
Time To	
With *family, friends etc*	
Near *other shoppers etc*	

Day	Date	Month	Year

Location shop, store etc	
Time From	
Time To	
With family, friends etc	
Near other shoppers etc	

Day	Date	Month	Year

Location shop, store etc	
Time From	
Time To	
With family, friends etc	
Near other shoppers etc	

Day	Date	Month	Year

Location shop, store etc	
Time From	
Time To	
With family, friends etc	
Near other shoppers etc	

Day	Date	Month	Year

Location *shop, store etc*	
Time From	
Time To	
With *family, friends etc*	
Near *other shoppers etc*	

Day	Date	Month	Year

Location *shop, store etc*	
Time From	
Time To	
With *family, friends etc*	
Near *other shoppers etc*	

Day	Date	Month	Year

Location *shop, store etc*	
Time From	
Time To	
With *family, friends etc*	
Near *other shoppers etc*	

Another Really Useful book...

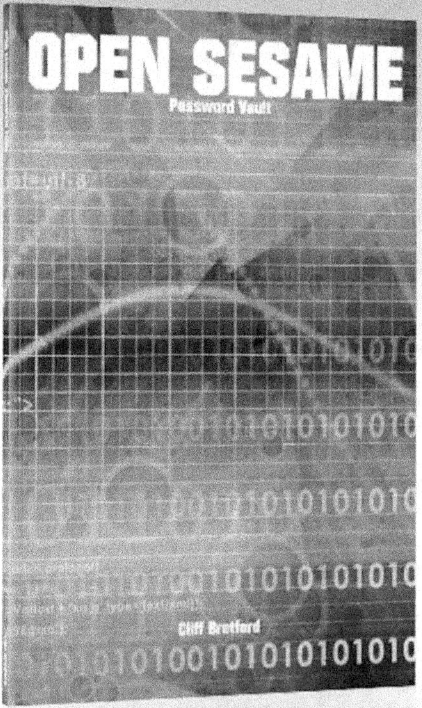

Nowadays, you need a password for just about everything you can think of - mobile phone, computer, Wi-Fi, email, social media and banking to name but a few. So unless you have a phenomenal memory for remembering passwords and other associated security details you will no doubt already be writing down your passwords or password prompts anyway, probably on scraps of paper or storing passwords in your email account

So instead of doing either of these, you can now write your password details down in this easy to use book. Disguised as a novel and containing some useful password tips, it has been clearly laid out in alphabetical order for ease of access, allowing you to record all your various security details.

Available now from all good book sellers!
ISBN: 978-1540443274